T0156349

BASIC HEALTH
PUBLICATIONS
USER'S GUIDE

TO SAW PALMETTO & MEN'S HEALTH

*Learn What You Need
to Know about
Reducing Your
Risk of Prostate
Disease.*

MICHAEL JANSON, M.D.

JACK CHALLEM Series Editor

The information contained in this book is based upon the research and personal and professional experiences of the author. It is not intended as a substitute for consulting with your physician or other healthcare provider. Any attempt to diagnose and treat an illness should be done under the direction of a healthcare professional.

The publisher does not advocate the use of any particular healthcare protocol but believes the information in this book should be available to the public. The publisher and author are not responsible for any adverse effects or consequences resulting from the use of the suggestions, preparations, or procedures discussed in this book. Should the reader have any questions concerning the appropriateness of any procedures or preparation mentioned, the author and the publisher strongly suggest consulting a professional healthcare advisor.

Series Editor: Jack Challem
Editor: Roberta W. Waddell
Typesetter: Gary A. Rosenberg
Series Cover Designer: Mike Stromberg

Basic Health Publications User's Guides are published by Basic Health Publications, Inc.

Copyright © 2002 by Michael Janson

ISBN: 978-1-59120-030-7 (Pbk.)
ISBN: 978-1-68162-873-8 (Hardcover)

CONTENTS

INTRODUCTION

Some dramatic changes have been taking place in Western medicine in the past few years, and you have the opportunity to benefit from some of these changes. Costs of healthcare have been skyrocketing, and the government and insurance companies have tried to implement some form of control on the costs by managing the way doctors treat patients. At the same time, there has been an explosive growth in demand for treatments that are less invasive than surgery and less risky than prescription medications.

Why the changes? Consider that prescription medications are the fourth or fifth leading cause of death in the United States, with more than 100,000 people dying every year from their side effects, even when taken correctly. Heart bypass surgery is the ninth leading cause of death. Safe alternatives to drugs and surgery are available for almost every condition that plagues our society, but most doctors are only just beginning to learn about them. While still resistant to change, the medical profession is starting to recognize the benefits of natural treatments to complement or even replace some conventional medical care.

When I finished medical school in 1970, I knew very little about nutrition. Although I did learn the basic biochemistry of the individual nutrients, I did not have any training in how that related to good nutrition and dietary habits, or how the nutrients could be used as dietary supplements for treatment of different medical conditions. I also had no information about herbs and botanicals, which had been the mainstay of medicine in this country before this century, and still contribute greatly to medical therapy in many countries.

The German government, recognizing the popularity and importance of herbs in medicine, established a commission (commission E) to look into botanical medicine and establish some standards by which doctors could understand how to use herbs as part of their medical practices. In Germany and other countries, a large number of general practitioners use these herbs routinely, but they have still not been accepted in the United States. A small percentage of doctors here have been using these treatments—including vitamins, minerals, amino acids, essential oils, accessory nutrients, and botanicals—for many years with great success.

Often, these doctors have been the objects of ridicule among their peers. They have also been the objects of disciplinary action by their medical boards, which regulate the practice of medicine in every state. Public demand, fortunately, has been forcing a change in this policy, and creating a more congenial atmosphere for innovative physicians. Many states have now passed legislation protecting doctors from these medical board actions, and making sure that patients have access to alternatives to drugs and surgery. A movement is underway to change federal regulations to accomplish this on a nationwide scale, and everyone will benefit from these changes (except perhaps some drug companies).

In addition to beneficial foods, vitamins, minerals, essential fatty acids, and amino acids, herbs and botanicals are important contributors to this resurgence in natural healthcare. One of the most valuable dietary supplements has been the botanical product derived from the berries of the saw palmetto tree. In addition to European doctors, physicians in the United States are recommending saw palmetto for the treatment of prostate disorders. This is based on its long history of use in folk medicine for the treatment of urinary tract disorders, and on the recent research supporting its value. The German commission, and even the United States Food and Drug Administration, have evaluated some of this information. The results of their investigations and their conclusions may surprise you.

The combination of research and clinical experience with saw palmetto gives you the opportunity to use this simple, safe, effective, and cost-effective dietary supplement to manage your prostate problems, and possibly avoid medication and surgery. However, saw palmetto is only a part of a complete program for prostate health, and prostate health is just one part of the overall picture of men's health. Functioning fully in every way, and maintaining that function for as long as possible as you age, is the end result of taking good care of yourself.

CHAPTER 1

THE PROSTATE GLAND IN MEN'S HEALTH

Almost everyone has heard about the prostate gland, but you may not know what it is or how it is important in health. As men age, it is almost certain that they will become intimately familiar with the details of their prostate gland, and possibly have to deal with it as a health issue. The more you know about your prostate, the easier it will be to understand how to help yourself or help your doctor understand the treatments you prefer.

Prostate Anatomy and Function

The prostate gland is a small organ found only in men that sits below and behind the bladder and above and in front of the rectum. It consists of a collection of ducts, fibrous tissue, glandular tissue, and muscle tissue, and it surrounds the urethra, which takes the urine from the bladder through the penis and out. The normal prostate is about the size of a walnut, weighs about two-thirds of an ounce (20 g), and produces prostatic fluids that combine with sperm from the testicles and other secretions to form semen. These fluids help sperm survive and improve their ability to travel (motility).

Urethra
A canal that takes the urine from the bladder, past the prostate, and out through the penis. Semen is also discharged through it.

The prostate also has some muscle fibers surrounding the urethra that help with urination. When they contract, they push urine out to aid in emptying the bladder. They also play a role during orgasm by pushing some of the prostate fluid and some of the sperm from the testicles into the urethra and out through the penis. Although it is very small, the strategic location of the prostate surrounding the urethra leads to far more health problems and medical care costs than would be predicted from its size alone.

Prostate
A small organ in men that sits below and behind the bladder and produces prostatic fluids that help form semen.

Prostate Problems with Aging

One of the most common, and problematic, changes in the prostate results from its gradual enlargement with age (benign enlargement, not a cancer). This enlargement eventually leads to compression of the urethra and restriction of the urine flow. It is called benign prostatic hyperplasia (or hypertrophy—an older term that is still used), abbreviated as BPH. In addition to the direct obstruction that enlargement causes (the mechanical or static component of BPH), the muscles and nerves of the prostate, bladder outlet, and urethra can contribute further to the symptoms (the dynamic component).

Hyperplasia
Increased growth of cells of any kind, leading to enlargement of the organ. Also known as hypertrophy in reference to the prostate.

Prostate problems are very common, indeed. More than 50 percent of men over age forty have enlarged prostate glands. By the time they reach eighty years old, 80 to 90 percent of men have an enlarged prostate. Although surgery to remove some of the prostate tissue is a common procedure for benign enlargement, it is not always necessary; only about 10 percent of men end up having prostate surgery at some time in their lives. According to a 1996 study, enlarged prostates lead to about $4 billion in healthcare expenditures.

There are also other possible problems with the prostate. It can be inflamed as a result of infection with bacteria, or even more frequently, with other organisms, leading to local aching, pain and burning on urination, testicular discomfort, and low back pain, as well as white blood cells in the prostatic secretions and urine. This prostate inflammation, or prostatitis, can be acute or chronic. It is even possible to see these symptoms with no signs of inflammation (no white blood cells in the prostatic secretions). In this situation, the symptoms are referred to as prostatodynia. These prostate ailments are not related to age, and are commonly seen in younger men.

The prostate is also subject to cellular changes that lead to cancer, the most common cancer in men. Prostate cancers are often undiagnosed, and only found in an autopsy when a man dies from other causes. As with many other cancers, diet may play a significant role in the development of prostate cancer.

The Symptoms of Prostate Enlargement

Benign prostatic hyperplasia (BPH) leads to a gradually increasing pinching of the urethra and obstruction of the urine flow. The early symptoms may simply start with reduction of the size and force of the urine stream. Young men with normal prostates have

BPH
Benign prostatic hyperplasia (or hyper-trophy). Enlargement of the prostate that leads to a pinching off of the urethra.

a peak urine flow of about two-thirds of an ounce (20 ml) per second or higher. This normally declines somewhat with age, but even more so with BPH. With mild BPH, the peak flow is reduced to approximately one-half ounce (15–20 ml) per second. With moderate prostate enlargement, the flow rate drops to between one-third and one-half ounce (10–15 ml) per second, and with severe BPH the peak rate is below one-third ounce (10 ml) per second. Severe obstruction of the urine flow can lead to serious kidney disease.

The urine flow may be difficult to start; a symptom called hesitancy. This delay in starting urination usually requires some pushing or straining in order to begin the urine flow. Because the bladder muscles help get the last bit of urine out, if there is an obstruction in your urethra, these muscles will have a harder time emptying your bladder completely (because they compensate for this by getting stronger, the symptoms of BPH may not appear early on). As a result of this difficulty, every time you urinate, some residual urine will be left in the bladder, which can give you the feeling that you have not finished emptying your bladder (another sign of prostate enlargement), and this constant feeling makes you want to urinate more frequently.

One of the most upsetting symptoms of BPH is frequent nighttime urination. Often, men with prostate enlargement may have to get up two, three, even six or more times at night to try to empty their bladder. This is obviously very disturbing to sleep, which is often already a problem for people as they get older. This nighttime urination is caused by a combination of urine left in the bladder, irritation of the urethra, and changes in the functioning of the kidneys.

Other Symptoms of Prostate Enlargement

The standard evaluation of a man with prostate enlargement includes estimating the severity of the problem. For example, being unable to hold in the urine or having difficulty postponing urination is called urgency—the sense that you have to go and can't wait. Sometimes there is interrupted stream, or intermittency where the urine flow will stop in the middle and the muscles have to strain to start again.

When there is very little urine in the bladder and the urge to urinate arises, this could be due to changes in the bladder, prostate, and urethra. With the prostate enlarged, the straining needed to start urinating, and the increased amount of work for the muscles of the bladder and prostate, there may be an irritation in the area of the bladder where the urethra starts, or in the part of the urethra that runs through the prostate. The irritation increases the sense of urgency and, therefore, the frequency of urination, but it is unrelated to the actual amount of urine present. This irritation of the urethra and the muscle spasms it causes in the bladder and prostate result in uncomfortable, sometimes painful urination, a symptom called dysuria.

Dysuria
Pain or discomfort on urination that results from irritation of the urethra and spasms of the bladder and prostate muscles.

Evaluating the Severity of Prostate Enlargement

In addition to physical examinations, for many years doctors have used a questionnaire called the Boyarsky Index where patients evaluate the level of nine symptoms on a scale from zero (not present) to three (most severe) for a maximum symptom score of twenty-seven. Another scale, the American Urological Association Symptom Index, uses six symptoms, rated from zero to five, plus the nighttime urinary frequency. In this scale, a score up to seven is mild, up to eighteen is moderate, and above nineteen is considered a severe prostate disorder (prostatism).

These, along with other scores and the examination, help evaluate the prostate symptoms, and are used to determine how much improvement there is with any treatment.

Finding Out if You Have a Prostate Problem

Generally, symptoms appear early in the course of benign prostate enlargement, but they can vary a great deal. Even with moderate BPH, the symptoms may be minimal because the bladder muscle can grow to compensate for the obstruction. And the telltale symptoms of more frequent, more urgent, or nighttime urination may be caused by something else entirely, such as anxiety, caffeine consumption, or drinking large amounts of liquid.

After age forty, it's a good idea to have annual checkups to detect the presence or ongoing development of BPH. This normally includes a digital rectal examination (DRE), in which a doctor places a gloved finger in the rectum to evaluate the size and shape of the prostate gland. This exam does not always give the full picture, so other tests are also done, including one that measures the rate of flow of the urine, ultrasound studies, and magnetic resonance imaging (MRI).

Differentiating Benign Prostate Enlargement from Cancer

Benign enlargement is far more prevalent than

cancer, but cancer is certainly common enough to be of concern. Cancers produce hard, rough, irregular lumps, or nodules, but with benign enlargement, the prostate is usually softer, smoother, and more even. This can vary, however—the cancer nodules could be buried deep within the prostate, for example, and the doctor's gloved finger would not be able to reach them so they would remain undetected in a physical examination.

There is also the prostate specific antigen test (PSA), which tests for a specific substance found in larger amounts in the blood of patients with prostate cancer. It is not foolproof in distinguishing prostate cancer from BPH or prostatitis, but it can help. The amount of the protein molecule PSA in the blood rises when prostate cells grow or are inflamed. Since cancer cells tend to grow more vigorously than other prostate cells, the level of PSA is likely to be much higher with prostate cancer than with other conditions. The PSA will, however, also be higher for a day or two after ejaculation, so it is important to give the doctor this information when taking this test.

Prostate Specific Antigen

A protein molecule produced by prostate cells and found in the blood. In increased levels, it may indicate prostate cancer.

Other Diagnostic Tests

Another test is an ultrasound of the prostate done through the rectum. Ultrasound tests are not dangerous. They are used all the time to evaluate hidden body structures and, in pregnancy, to evaluate the developing fetus. Sound waves are reflected off of tissue, and they give a picture of the prostate, which can indicate its size and the presence of lumps that can't be felt. This test is usually reserved for those who have had another positive test first.

Finally, a biopsy, where a tissue sample from a specific organ is taken, can be done on the prostate. It can be an open biopsy where a piece of tissue gets cut from the prostate, or it can be a needle biopsy, possible in this case because of the relatively easy access to the prostate gland through the rectum. With this kind of biopsy, a needle is inserted into the gland and a piece of tissue is taken for microscopic examination.

CHAPTER 2

CONVENTIONAL MEDICAL TREATMENT OF THE PROSTATE

For many years, the only treatment for benign prostatic hyperplasia was to wait until the symptoms were intolerable, or the urinary retention created a more serious medical problem. If the prostate is enlarged but no symptoms appear, waiting is not a problem as sometimes the prostate does not enlarge further or cause symptoms. On the other hand, if it does progress enough for symptoms to appear, then a doctor would recommend treatment.

Surgical removal of the obstructive prostate tissue is common. Today, several surgical options are available. Doctors can do an open operation, from the outside, but this is not a common procedure for BPH, although it may be used for cancer or when there are massively enlarged glands. The prostate tissue can also be removed through a tube (cystoscope) placed into the urethra through the penis. This procedure, called a transurethral resection of the prostate (TURP), removes the tissue right where the urinary obstruction occurs, and can be quite effective.

However, even though TURP is still the main treatment for the more severe situations, there can be complications, as for example, a retrograde ejaculation where the semen is pushed into the bladder rather than out through the penis. Sexual dysfunction or impotence, seen in one out of every ten to twenty patients, is another complication, as is incontinence. Some men develop a urinary tract infection after the surgery, which requires antibiotics, and sometimes they have excessive bleeding that requires blood transfusions. In one out of five or ten patients, a repeat operation is often required if the symptoms return.

Other Treatments for BPH

Newer, minimally invasive treatments have been developed and are still being studied, but they seem very promising as far as surgical procedures go. Called minimally invasive because, although they use a catheter to enter the urethra, they do not cut the prostate tissue. For example, in the transurethral needle ablation (TUNA) procedure, a catheter is used to insert into the prostate small needles that transmit low-level radio waves that create heat and destroy some prostate cells. This has fewer complications than TURP, but it does not appear quite as effective in the long term.

Another treatment is called transurethral microwave therapy (TUMT), which uses microwaves, also to create heat and destroy prostate tissue. So far, TUMT appears to require repeat procedures sooner than other therapies, making it less effective in the long term than other treatments. While none of these newer treatments are as effective as TURP, they *are* safer, less invasive, and have fewer side effects. They also take less time, are less expensive, and can be done in a doctor's office, usually with very rapid recovery.

More recently, two other procedures have been evaluated. One of these is treatment with a transurethral ultrasound-guided laser-induced prostatectomy (TULIP) device. It also destroys some prostate tissue, using ultrasound to direct a laser beam at the prostate tissue. As with the above, it has fewer side effects than conventional surgery.

The other very promising treatment is called transurethral vaporization of the prostate (TUVP). In this method, the prostate tissue is rapidly vaporized with high heat. In one three-year follow-up of this treatment, published in the *British Journal of Urology International,* the relief from symptoms was equivalent to the results with TURP. However, the complication rate was also about the same in the two groups.

When considering treatment, it is well to appreciate that any procedure has some associated risks, and no one wants surgical procedures if they can avoid them. No doctor recommends such treatments unless the symptoms are significant, but even when they do recommend them, alternatives without the risks of surgery would often be adequate.

Nonsurgical Prostate Treatments

Until recently, most conventional physicians have not had any treatments to offer to patients with prostate enlargement other than to wait until the symptoms worsened and surgery was required. In the mid-1990s, a new medication called finasteride (trade name Proscar) was shown to help with prostate symptoms, but it was not nearly as effective as doctors (and especially patients) had hoped it would be. It also turned out to have undesirable side effects, among them a loss of libido, sexual dysfunction (inability to have or maintain an erection, or impotence), and abnormal ejaculation. There is also a risk of birth defects to a male fetus in a pregnant woman who has contact with the drug, through handling either the pill or the semen of a man taking it.

Because of these potential side effects and the

drug's inadequate results, both doctors and patients would like to find other ways than finasteride to reduce BPH symptoms and delay or eliminate the need for surgery.

The Role of Enzymes and Hormones in BPH

Finasteride appears to work through its effects on hormones and an enzyme. Enzymes are protein molecules that act as catalysts—substances that make chemical reactions occur faster at body temperature. The rate of a reaction is determined by many factors, such as heat and the mixture of substances that are reacting. Because excessive heat might damage cells, enzyme catalysts help promote reactions at lower temperatures. Enzymes work with other substances, such as minerals and vitamins, to push these reactions. Many vitamins are called coenzymes because of their role in helping enzymes work.

Well-known examples of enzymes are the digestive enzymes, produced in the stomach and pancreas, which work with stomach acids to break down foods during digestion and help in their assimilation. Different kinds of enzymes also control the reactions that lead to the production of hormones and the reactions involved in the breakdown of hormones after they are used.

Hormones are regulatory substances produced by the endocrine glands. Unlike the output of other glands, such as sweat glands or salivary glands, they deliver their output directly into the bloodstream. Adrenaline (epinephrine), a well-known hormone, is produced by the adrenal glands in response to acute stress. Another hormone, cortisone, is produced by a different part of the adrenal glands. The pancreas produces insulin, a hormone that regulates blood sugar levels.

The thyroid gland in the neck is another endocrine gland. Thyroid hormones regulate the metabolic rate, or how fast your body burns energy.

At the base of the brain is the master endocrine gland, the pituitary, which produces substances that regulate other glands. It also produces hormones that have direct effects on different bodily functions. For example, it regulates the amounts of testosterone produced in the testes of men, and the amounts of estrogens and progesterone produced in the ovaries of women. Referred to as the male and female sex hormones, there are, in fact, small amounts of each found in the other sex as well.

Finasteride's Effect on Hormones

The male sex hormones, or androgens, are primarily testosterone and a derivative called dihydrotestosterone (DHT) produced from testosterone with the help of an enzyme called 5-alpha reductase. Finasteride works by blocking this enzyme to reduce the production of DHT, which has been shown to promote prostate enlargement. Therefore, blocking its production helps reduce prostate symptoms.

Hormones
Regulatory substances produced by the endocrine glands that control numerous functions in the body.

The hormone relationship is not quite so clear, however. In dogs, the female hormone estradiol (a relatively strong member of the estrogen family of hormones) acts together with the DHT to increase prostate growth, and it may also do so in men. Another enzyme, aromatase, converts some of the circulating testosterone into estradiol, which may contribute more to prostate enlargement than DHT does. Finasteride does not directly influence the production of estradiol, but there is speculation that its blocking the production of DHT may lead to more estradiol production, which can worsen prostate symptoms, and may be one of the reasons finasteride does not work as well as we would like.

The Causes of Benign Prostatic Hyperplasia

We don't completely understand the cause of benign prostate enlargement. We do know that it happens with aging and requires the presence of male hormones, specifically DHT, de-rived from testosterone. Men who have had their testicles removed, and therefore have no testosterone production, do not develop benign prostatic hyperplasia. And, in dogs, we know that hormonal therapy, which increases DHT levels, leads to an enlargement of the prostate similar to BPH.

Dihydro-testosterone (DHT) *A hormone derived from testosterone, the male sex hormone that is an apparent cause of benign prostate enlargement.*

In addition, as men age, the level of the estrogen hormone estradiol increases. As we said, in dogs, estradiol works with DHT to induce prostate growth. If this happens in humans also, it might explain the increase in prostate size with aging because, as men age, their DHT level goes down, but their estradiol level goes up. Some researchers also suggest that the ratio of DHT to testosterone, which goes up with age, is more important than the absolute level of either one.

Lifestyle choices may play a role in the development of BPH, and improper nutrition may contribute not only to prostate enlargement, but also to prostate cancer. It is also possible that specific beneficial foods may contribute to the prevention of prostate enlargement.

Other Medical Treatments for BPH

Doctors may prescribe another drug that helps with the symptoms of prostate enlargement. This drug terazosin (Hytrin) has been used for high blood pressure because it relaxes the muscles of the blood vessels, allowing them to open and reduce the pressure in the circulation. Terazosin works to improve urine flow but does not affect the size of the prostate. Unfortunately, as with most medications, there are some potential side effects from terazosin. Because it is also a blood pressure medication, one major caution is that the first dose of terazosin may cause very low blood pressure and fainting in the first few days of taking it, or you could momentarily feel faint when you stand up quickly. It can also cause dizziness, fatigue, sleepiness, and sexual dysfunction as well as nasal congestion and a runny nose. If you also have high blood pressure, you may have other side effects, and if you are on other blood pressure medications, be sure to let your doctor know before taking terazosin.

CHAPTER 3

SAW PALMETTO: THE MEN'S HERB

Dietary supplements, including herbs and botanicals, are becoming more popular as treatments for common medical conditions, partly because they usually have the advantage over drugs and surgery of being safer, more cost effective, and less invasive. In many cases, they are not only safer and less expensive, but they are also more effective than some drugs prescribed for the same conditions. There are supplements for the brain, digestion, the heart, the liver, and the skin, as well as for arthritis, diabetes, headaches, and many other conditions. Saw palmetto is one of the supplements that is not only cheaper, but more effective than the medications used for the prostate.

Saw Palmetto Compared to Drugs

It is likely that most men will have to consider dealing with their own prostate as they age. If it does become a problem for you, you have the choices listed above for treatment, or you may wish to choose an alternative that has numerous advantages over the drugs/surgery treatments used by conventional medicine. It is no secret that most people would prefer to avoid surgery if possible, especially men contemplating surgery on their prostate gland.

Based on the medical literature, my own use of

it with my patients, and the experience of most of my colleagues in nutritional and botanical medicine, saw palmetto is a safe, effective alternative to these treatments. Even some urologists who have been disappointed with finasteride are recommending saw palmetto instead. It reduces the symptoms of prostate enlargement, and it also helps improve urinary tract function in a large percentage of men with benign prostatic hyperplasia (BPH). You might also consider taking saw palmetto as preventive medicine if you are in the age group at risk for BPH.

What Is Saw Palmetto?

The saw palmetto is a small palm tree eight to ten feet high that grows in the southeastern coastal states of North America. The tree has large, fan-like leaves, and produces berries about the size of a grape that have a deep reddish-black to brown color. These berries have long been used for disorders of the urinary tract, especially by Native Americans. Saw palmetto is also known as Sabal serrulata, Serenoa repens, or by its trade name Permixon.

Saw Palmetto
A small palm tree with red-brown berries that have been researched in Europe and the United States for treating disorders of the prostate gland.

Recent European research on the oily, fat-soluble extracts of saw palmetto berries has shown their benefits in treating disorders of the prostate gland. Most of this research comes from France and Germany, where the use of botanical medicines is more accepted and better researched than in the United States. This is slowly changing, however, as North Americans have developed a strong interest in alternatives to drugs and surgery, and have opened their minds to nutrition and dietary supplements, including botanical medicines. Research is now being done in the United States, England, Scotland, Russia, Italy, and elsewhere.

Botanical Medicines

Botanical medicine is the use of any plant parts in treating or preventing illness. Doctors or other healers might use different parts of certain plants. Technically, herbs are the leafy or stem parts of the plant, but when used in medicinal treatments, the word "herb" often means botanical, referring to any part of the plant—the bark, fruit, leaf, rhizome, root, or stem. Many botanical medicines are at the root of our modern drugs, such as digitalis, for the heart, which comes from the leaf of the foxglove, or colchicine, for gout, from the bulb of the autumn crocus. And aspirin is a derivative of salicylic acid, a substance that comes from willow bark.

The prescription medications that doctors commonly use for treatment of illness are often quite risky. Side effects are common, and can be serious, sometimes leading to hospitalization and even death. Even over-the-counter medications frequently have side effects, so it is no wonder people are looking for safer, more natural remedies for their health problems. Most of the time, botanical medicines are safer than more recently developed medicines, but that does not mean they are all without risk. Saw palmetto is a very safe herb, and is one of several natural treatments for prostate disorders.

Botanical Medicine

Any therapeutic natural substance, commonly called an herb, derived from any part of a plant, usually with few or no toxic side effects.

Saw Palmetto and Prostate Treatment

For a number of years, practitioners who use nutrition and botanical medicines have had several alternative treatments for prostate enlargement not commonly used by conventional medicine, especially in the United States. High doses of zinc, for example, have been shown to help with the symptoms of BPH, as have essential fatty acids and high doses of certain amino acids (amino acids are the building blocks of proteins) when taken as supplements.

As mentioned above, saw palmetto can have a profound effect in providing relief from the symptoms of BPH, even better than the results seen with finasteride, and without its troubling side effects. While saw palmetto may also act as an inhibitor of the enzyme 5-alpha reductase, thus reducing the DHT production thought to enlarge the prostate, it appears to have other physiological effects as well that make it superior to the medication. This is especially true because of its lack of side effects.

For example, saw palmetto extracts inhibit all of the testosterone, not just DHT, and unlike finasteride, which only acts on certain cells, the extracts work in all of the cells studied, helping to prevent prostate enlargement.

Studies on saw palmetto show that it improves both the rate and the volume of urine flow. It reduces the urgency and frequency of urination, including the number of urinations at night. Overall, about 90 percent of men report that it helps them with their symptoms compared to finasteride (which helps only about 50 percent of them, does not decrease nighttime urination, has minimal effect on urine flow, and has side effects!)

Other Effects of Saw Palmetto on the Prostate

Research shows there are other physiological effects of saw palmetto that help prostate symptoms, and may help other medical conditions as well. It can inhibit certain substances called pros - tanoids that lead to inflammation, irritation, and smooth muscle spasms, among other symptoms. Some of them promote inflammation while others decrease it, and any imbalance among the different types can lead to significant health problems.

These processes influence the symptoms of prostate enlargement, and saw palmetto can help reduce them, and minimize the irritation and spasm of the smooth muscles in the prostate and urethra that initiate the urgency and frequency of BPH. Research confirms that saw palmetto has these additional benefits for BPH, beyond its effect on DHT and the size of the prostate. So if you have prostate symptoms, you can get the benefits of both finasteride and terazosin from saw palmetto extracts without the risk of their side effects.

Saw Palmetto also Affects Estrogens

In addition to testosterone, men produce some female estrogen hormones (although less than women), just as women produce some testosterone. Receptors are the locations where the hormones bind to cells to have their ultimate effects, just as a key fits into a lock in order to turn it. You can influence the activity of a hormone without changing the amount that is produced if you change the number of receptors, or the ability of the hormone to attach to the receptor. Instead of inhibiting the production of the estrogen hormones, saw palmetto takes over the same receptor sites

Estrogens
A group of hormones found in high amounts in women, and far lower amounts in men, that influence reproductive organs and other body functions.

as the estrogen, and works on both kinds of these estrogen receptor sites to reduce the activity of estradiol, which otherwise increases the symptoms of BPH (not to mention its potential for increasing the risk of prostate cancer). So, saw palmetto reduces BPH symptoms that way also.

Prostate Symptoms Vary from Time to Time

From hour to hour, or day to day, the intensity of prostate symptoms can vary, with stress contributing to the symptoms. For example, everyone has had the experience of having a strong urge to urinate, but before finding a bathroom the urge has diminished greatly or even disappeared. This is because the signals from the nerves of the urethra and bladder are variable. But stress can increase the sense of urgency, as can the sound of running water, or alcohol, caffeine, and any food sensitivities. Muscle spasms in the bladder, prostate, and urethra can also lead to a feeling of urgency and to more frequent urination. For these reasons, the urge to urinate can come and go, even when the amount of urine in the bladder is unchanged, and in spite of the size of the prostate.

In fact, in a large percentage of men, symptoms improve with no treatment, even though there is no change in the size of the prostate. Eventually, as the prostate enlarges with age, the symptoms will be more consistent, but in the meantime, this variation is common and expected.

CHAPTER 4

PROSTATE RESEARCH: HOW IS IT DONE?

First, let me give you some information about medical research, so you can understand the studies on saw palmetto and drugs. Medical research varies greatly in quality and consistency, and for many reasons, any one study must be viewed with caution, especially if it is contrary to a number of other studies. The methods and design play a large role in determining the outcome, and the position of the authors strongly influences the interpretation and conclusions, and the way studies are reported. Even established journals may publish studies that are of inferior quality, but that does not mean the research is valueless. It may stimulate other studies and provide some good information, even if not all of it is valid.

Understanding the Placebo Effect

When doctors do medical research, they are always on the lookout for effects that may appear to be due to a treatment, but in reality are due to other factors. This is particularly the case when symptoms of an illness are variable and affected by stress or emotions. It is also an important consideration when the signs of an illness are subjective (reported by the patient) rather than objective (measured by a lab test or other equipment).

Symptoms are also affected by the expectations of the test subject and even the person ad-

ministering the test, so medical researchers intro-
duce controls to their studies to find out if the
results are due to these expectations. *Placebo*
comes from the Latin word meaning "to please"—
the patients trying to please
the doctor by reporting that
their symptoms are better as a
result of the doctor's treatment.
The symptoms may actually be
better, because we know that
the brain has a strong influence
on the healing process, but the
symptoms may not be influ-
enced by the treatment, which is what the study
is trying to determine. This is what is meant by
the placebo effect.

Placebo Effect
*Any benefit that is
due to a patient's expec-
tation of improvement
from a treatment, rather
than from the specific
treatment being
administered.*

Placebos in Practice

When doing a study, doctors will use a dummy
pill, the placebo, in half the test subjects. The
other half will get a real medicine that the doctors
are trying to test. The placebo, formerly called a
sugar pill, should look exactly like the real treatment, and is supposed to be completely inactive
so the results of the study are not influenced by
any physiological effect (sometimes the dummy
pill unexpectedly turns out to be active, casting
doubt on the results of the study). The group receiving the placebo is called the control group.
The groups should be randomly selected (to
avoid prejudice during selection) and carefully
matched in every other way to increase the valid-
ity of the study.

The subjects in the study are not told what pill
they are getting. If that is the only hidden information, it is called a single-blind study. If, in addition, those administering the pills do not know
which group is receiving which pill (they are

coded for later interpretation), it is called a "double-blind" study. In crossover studies, the groups are switched after a period of time, so the placebo group is given the real pill and the active-treatment group is given the placebo. (There are problems with some crossover studies because, if the active ingredients have long-lasting effects and the effects don't start right away, this confuses the outcome of the study.) Studies that test behavior or stress, instead of medication or some other substance, can also be conducted in a double-blind fashion, but they are more difficult to do.

Placebo-Controlled Studies Are Important for Prostate Research

Stress, the emotional state, or the person's expectations of the treatment's benefits often influence prostate symptoms. The dynamic component of these symptoms relates to spasms of the local muscles and irritation of the nerves and mucous membranes lining the bladder and urethra, and these dynamic symptoms are particularly influenced by the mind. Reactions, such as your hands sweating or becoming cold when you are nervous, are everyday evidence of the mind's influence on physical symptoms. Mind-body medicine, referring to harnessing the power of the mind to promote healing, is another bit of evidence showing how important your emotional and mental states are in any disease.

Studies designed to show that the effect of a particular treatment is due to the treatment itself, rather than the mind-body influence, need placebo controls in order for researchers to draw accurate conclusions. Although such controlled studies are not the only way to learn about the value of a treatment, establishment doctors do like to see them before accepting a treatment, especially one that is not typically part of conventional medicine. Fortunately, many nutritional and herbal treatments have controlled studies to support their value. Saw palmetto has been researched in a number of double-blind, placebo-controlled studies, many of them from France, Germany, and Italy.

Research on Saw Palmetto and Prostate Symptoms

Quite a few of the studies showing how saw palmetto works have been published in recognized medical journals. There are human studies, animal studies, and studies of cells in laboratories, the latter designed to show how a substance works—show which biochemical and hormonal actions explain the results when the substance is given to a person. Skeptical scientists like to have some understanding of how something might work to show whether it really does work. Of course, this is not always possible. Many beneficial treatments are valuable, even though we have little understanding of their mechanisms. For many years, medical science did not have an explanation of how aspirin worked, but this did not stop doctors from recommending it. Many treatments today are in a similar situation. Cholesterol-lowering drugs, for example, have actions that are too quick to be related only to their effect on cholesterol. Researchers are now trying to find out if this is due to their effects on platelets or inflammation, or some other action.

Studies in cells have shown some of the actions of saw palmetto. Although we are not sure if the effects we see in cells in the lab are the ones responsible for the actual results when people take saw palmetto, it is likely that they are related.

Specific Studies and Their Results

The earliest study that I can find, from 1969, is a description of a substance in saw palmetto that has an estrogenlike effect. Fourteen years later, in 1983, a cell study showed that saw palmetto extract affected the testosterone receptors in rat prostate cells.

The first human study I could find was done in Germany in 1979. Seventy-four men were treated with an extract of Sabal serrulata (another name for saw palmetto). In this study they showed that, although the objective measurements of the prostate and urine flow did not change, every patient reported a reduction of their symptoms.

Another early human study was done by a French team in 1984. These researchers also reported the favorable results of a double-blind study using saw palmetto in 110 patients with BPH. A number of other studies since have shown similar results. One in Spain, in 1992, compared saw palmetto with a drug similar to terazosin, and both substances were found to be about equally effective.

A 1995 study done in Italy showed that saw palmetto was beneficial, but not quite as effective as another drug similar to terazosin. This is important for doctors and the public to know, because if they have a choice, most people would prefer to take a natural substance that is almost as effective and has fewer side effects, especially if it is less expensive. If it turns out the natural treatment doesn't control the symptoms, the person can always then take the medication.

Other Studies and United States Research

A New Zealand study showed saw palmetto and finasteride were similarly effective. The test subjects all had significant improvement in nighttime urination, daytime frequency of urination, and peak urine flow rates. In two large uncontrolled trials, about 90 percent of those studied reported that their symptoms were much better within three months after starting saw palmetto.

Some American doctors only trust studies done in the United States, not a reasonable prejudice because studies done in Italy, Germany, France, Spain, and elsewhere are just as valid as those done in the United States. Although most studies have been done abroad, in 1998 there was a study done in Chicago to evaluate saw palmetto for its effectiveness in treating prostate enlargement. After six months, they found that about half the people reported they had at least a 50 percent improvement in symptoms.

The FDA Evaluation of Saw Palmetto Research

The United States Food and Drug Administration (FDA) evaluated saw palmetto research in response to a request by one company that wanted to make a health claim for the effectiveness of their product on the label. Interestingly, this FDA evaluation came shortly after the prescription drug finasteride was approved. A number of the studies mentioned above were submitted for the FDA review. In their analysis, the FDA looked at these and published their conclusions in *Food Drug Cosmetic Law Reports*. After noting that the saw palmetto extract appeared to be safe, they evaluated nighttime urination frequency, urinary output, and residual urine, as well as the patients' reports on improvement of their discomfort while urinating. They reported that the urine-flow rate increased and the residual volume (the amount left in the bladder after urination) decreased, as did the nighttime urinations. They also noted that more than 92 percent of the patients reported that their symptoms were better.

These changes, the FDA admitted, were statistically significant. However, they went on to say that they did not consider these improvements to be clinically significant because the symptoms were not completely cured, even though in every case they were better than the already-approved drug. Over 90 percent of the patients reported they were better with saw palmetto, while only 50 percent did so with finasteride. The urine flow improved 50 percent with saw palmetto, compared to only 22 percent with finasteride. With saw palmetto, residual urine volume went down compared to no change with finasteride. *The Physicians' Desk Reference*, a guide to drugs that every physician uses, states that most patients report at least a 30 percent improvement with finasteride. This is *less* than in any of the studies I have seen with saw palmetto.

The FDA Conclusions: Did They Approve Saw Palmetto Claims?

In spite of their favorable review of the effects of saw palmetto, the FDA has not yet approved the use of saw palmetto for the prostate, but this has to be understood in context. It would be very unusual for the FDA to approve any natural substance in the treatment of medical conditions. Their official role is to assure the safety and promote the development of new drugs. In spite of that, many drugs that reach the market are neither safe nor effective, and are eventually pulled from the market (examples are thalidomide, Fen-phen, and Baycol), usually after they have done damage.

Drug companies pour enormous amounts of money into research and development to meet the standards of the FDA. But this is not a guarantee of safety or effectiveness. Most natural products on the market today have a long history of safety, but do not have the expensive studies that meet the FDA standards. This is because natural products cannot be patented, so the drug companies have no incentive to spend the money to meet those standards.

The FDA has an apparent bias against natural products like saw palmetto. Even when they do meet the standards, the FDA seems to find some excuse not to approve them. As mentioned above, the FDA found that saw palmetto produced better results than the prostate drug that they had already approved, but they still did not approve label claims for saw palmetto. The fact that the FDA has not approved saw palmetto says more about them than about this remarkable supplement, and in no way detracts from its value.

Doctors Recommend Saw Palmetto

Along with many of my medical colleagues, I regularly recommend the use of saw palmetto, but most doctors here are unfamiliar with herbal or nutritional medicine, and do not recommend it. This is beginning to change, however, as increasing numbers of urologists are starting to suggest it. Naturopaths and nutritionists, of course, have an interest in alternatives to drugs and surgery, and they regularly recommend saw palmetto for prostate enlargement.

In America, conventional doctors are often opposed to using herbal treatments or other dietary supplements, and doctors who do start using such treatments are no longer considered conventional, but this is not true in many other countries. In Germany, for example, about half of the primary doctors routinely use these treatments.

And in Italy in 1991, herbal treatments represented almost 10 percent of all prescriptions for prostate enlargement.

As increasing numbers of doctors are dissatisfied with the available drug treatments, and as their patients continue to demand more natural remedies, the number of conventional doctors who begin to use saw palmetto and other natural treatments will expand even further.

Natural Treatments May Take Time to Work

Saw palmetto takes some time to be effective in relieving the symptoms of prostate enlargement. Many people are used to medications having an instant effect to help with medical conditions, but this is not usually true for natural remedies. In the first few weeks of treatment, terazosin and similar drugs have been shown to be somewhat better at providing relief than saw palmetto, but longer studies show that saw palmetto eventually catches up with and surpasses these drugs.

Although some will report symptom relief sooner, typically you need to take saw palmetto for one to three months before significant results can be expected. In some studies, it appears that results are even better if those studied continue taking the saw palmetto for six months or more. In the Chicago study, one-fifth of the men were better after two months, one-third were better after four months, and nearly half were better after six months. Since they ended the study at that point, we don't know if any of the men would have had even further improvement with longer treatment. Of course, for those who do not respond adequately, it may help to take a larger dose, which might speed up and enhance the response.

Clinical Experience with Saw Palmetto

I have been treating my patients with saw palmetto for a number of years now. In my experience, patients usually tell me their symptoms have improved within two to three months, but sometimes sooner, even within a week or two. Occasionally, they tell me their symptoms persist. For them, it either takes much longer to see improvement, or they need a higher dose.

Very few fail to respond, at least to some extent, to saw palmetto, especially if they are given higher doses. For those few who don't, or for those with a more advanced disease, I recommend additional supplements, as you will see later. I have been very impressed with the success of this treatment. There have not been any serious side effects from it, in fact, almost no side effects at all. I myself am taking saw palmetto preventively as I approach sixty, even though I have never had any symptoms of prostate enlargement and have no evidence of it.

CHAPTER 5

GUIDELINES FOR BUYING AND USING SAW PALMETTO

Just learning about a supplement is not enough if you really want to use it for your health. You really need to know how to take it, what the precautions are, if any, what dose to use, and how it is available. You also need to know what to look for in products, so you are sure to get what will be most effective for you. I always give my patients specific instructions, and you need the same information.

Proper Dosing of Saw Palmetto

The typical recommended dose for most men with prostatic enlargement is 160 mg twice a day of the standardized extract, which contains 85 to 95 percent sterols and fatty acids. Most saw palmetto research is done with this daily dose of 320 mg, but if this is not effective, some men might benefit from higher doses. Responses are always variable with any medical treatment, especially natural substances, and we have to be prepared to make adjustments for individuals.

I had one eighty-seven-year-old man who was taking 320 mg of saw palmetto daily, and he reported it gave him only minimal, sporadic success in relieving his symptoms. Before giving up, after almost three years of disappointment, he decided to double his usual dose for a while. To his delight, after just one month, he reported back

that his symptoms were almost completely controlled. From having to get up and urinate three
to four times a night, he now only has to get up
once, or sometimes not at all. Needless to say, he
is staying on the 320 mg, twice-a-day dosage.

Timing the Doses of Saw Palmetto

Unlike some supplements, there is no special time
that will make saw palmetto more or less effective. The most convenient times to take dietary
supplements are with your breakfast and dinner.
Since supplements are basically foods, taking
them with meals usually helps to avoid any digestive upset that might occur with concentrated
food products. Also, since there are usually some
oils in foods, these may help absorb the fatty
substances in saw palmetto.

Although you could take your entire daily dose
at once, I usually recommend dividing the dose in
two. Taking it more than twice a day, however,
often results in forgetting the other doses, and
any supplement you don't take is going to be to-
tally ineffective. If you don't eat breakfast (although it is a good idea to do so), you can take
saw palmetto with lunch and dinner, along with
your other supplements, or you can take it all in
the evening. It's your choice; just don't forget to
take it.

Available Forms of Saw Palmetto

As with many botanical and herbal treatments, a
number of preparations are available. There are
whole berries, powders made from whole berries,
liquid extracts, such as concentrates, standardized extracts, and tinctures. Almost any of the
preparations will have some benefit, as long as
they honestly contain what is claimed on the
label. However, the dose needed to be effective

may vary greatly from one brand to another, and from one form to another.

Tinctures are extracts in a base of alcohol. You usually take a dropperful or two twice a day, unless otherwise instructed on the label. Some liquid extracts are in a glycerin base for people who prefer to avoid any alcohol. Liquid extracts can be effective if you take enough for your needs.

The dose of the berry powders will exceed the one for the extracts, and the most effective form is the standardized extract. Both the powders and the standardized extracts are available in either tablets or capsules. Some people find capsules easier to swallow, but manufacturers can fit more of the raw material into a tablet because it is compressed, and therefore smaller than the comparable dose in a capsule. Most of the time I have seen them in capsules. Read the dose carefully, as some products contain less than the usual 160 mg per pill. There are a number of these products on the market, and you just have to find what works for you.

Standardized Herbal Extracts

As our knowledge of botanical medicines advances, we are learning to identify the active substances in them that are therapeutic. We are able to research botanicals more easily if we can be sure that the amount of the active substance is consistent from batch to batch. Standardization means that the presumed active principles are always present in the same amount. Most of the standardized extracts have fairly reliable amounts of all the potential active components. In addition, it is a good idea to choose products that have at least some of the whole herb in them.

Most of the recent research on botanical medicines has been done with standardized extracts because they are the most reliable scientifically based herbs. Remember, however, that before there were standardized extracts, herbs had been used therapeutically for many centuries, and simple herbal preparations are still of value. Still, if you want the most reliable form of an herb, it is probably best to choose the standardized extracts as they have the known amounts of active components.

Getting the Right Product

If a product contains the standardized extract, it should say so on the label. It should also specify that it is standardized to contain 85 to 95 percent liposterols right on the ingredient label. If it simply says "extract" or "concentrate," or any other wording, it is probably not the standardized extract. This does not mean you may not get some value from it, only that it has not been as extensively researched. Most pills on the market contain 120 or 160 mg, so you can take two or three to get the recommended amount.

Standardized Extract
An herbal medicine that contains specific amounts of active components based on the current state of research.

It is also a good idea to look at the price of a few products (making sure that the doses are comparable). Occasionally, a product will be misbranded, and will not contain what the label says, but this is not the usual situation. As the supplement industry has matured, only a few disreputable companies may be cutting corners and charging less for their inferior products. If you compare prices for different high-quality brands at several health food stores and mail-order sources, you should have some idea of the usual price range for saw palmetto (as well as for any other health product you buy). If a product is far above or below the average price, be suspicious—on the high end, that you're not receiving value for your money, and on the low end, that you're not getting the right product. Good quality brands do, of course, go on special sale at a very good price from time to time, but that is usually a temporary deal.

Taking Saw Palmetto: How Long?

If saw palmetto is working, you will probably have to continue taking it indefinitely. Prostate enlargement is a progressive condition that generally worsens with age, and if you stop taking the treatment, the condition will gradually return. For some of the symptoms, the effect of saw palmetto is short term, and they may come back within a short time if you stop taking the supplement.

We don't really have any long-term studies to show what happens after someone improves with saw palmetto, then stops taking it, but we know from anecdotal experience that the hormonal changes from saw palmetto continue for only a short time after stopping the treatment. So basically, since there are no side effects to saw palmetto, it's a good idea to continue taking it in order to maintain your prostate health and control the symptoms of BPH.

Tolerance to the Effects of Saw Palmetto

In studies lasting up to twelve months, it was found that the benefits of taking saw palmetto do not decline if you continue taking it for the long term. The improvement in symptoms is maintained, and you do not develop a tolerance to it, meaning that the dose you need to maintain the benefits does not have to be increased. In fact, it appears that at the same dosage, the benefits continue to *increase* for the entire duration of the longer studies.

Although I have not seen any studies longer than one year, from the available research, my own clinical experience, and that of my colleagues, it seems the effects of saw palmetto last well beyond the duration of the longest studies.

Side Effects from Saw Palmetto

As previously stated, there are almost no side effects from saw palmetto, even in the higher doses. Of course, any substance, even water, given in extremely large quantities may have some negative effects, so it is probably best not to take more than twice the recommended amount. Approximately 5 percent of those studied have reported side effects, such as minor indigestion that does not last, but they're not usually enough for them to stop taking saw palmetto. In my own practice, only a few have reported digestive upset, and it was never clear that this was related to saw palmetto.

Saw palmetto has no contraindications (medical language for special medical situations in which you should not take a substance). There are also no known negative interactions with drugs or other dietary supplements. In fact, other dietary supplements and natural treatments may help relieve the symptoms of prostate enlargement, and these often enhance the action of the saw palmetto.

I have not seen any studies on people taking saw palmetto along with either terazosin (Hytrin) or finasteride (Proscar). Most of the time, people take either the drug or the natural supplement, and it is probably best to choose between them, although harmful side effects are still unlikely, even if you combine saw palmetto with either of these drugs.

Saw Palmetto for Younger Men

Since saw palmetto has no contraindications, no significant side effects, and no known negative interactions with drugs or other dietary supplements, you should have no reason to worry about taking it, no matter how old you are. If you are under forty, I see no reason to take saw palmetto unless there is some specific reason for it. If there is, you can rest assured that it will not interfere with your stamina or endurance, and it will not affect your exercise program. The same holds true for older people.

Saw Palmetto and Side Benefits

As with many herbs and dietary supplements, there may be some unexpected effects. Unlike drugs, however, where the side effects are almost invariably negative, with vitamins, minerals, flavonoids, fatty acids, and other dietary supplements, there are often side benefits—unexpected effects that are beneficial. But this is not always the case, so if you have an unexpected negative reaction, you should stop taking any supplement and consult a doctor, preferably one knowledgeable about alternative and complementary medicine. You may only need to stop for a while, then start again, to learn that the negative reactions were unrelated to the supplement.

With saw palmetto, you may see other benefits for the urinary tract, or experience its historical usefulness in treating inflammation and respiratory symptoms, and its effectiveness as a mild sedative. Women have also taken it successfully for bladder and urinary tract health.

Saw Palmetto and Drugs

Saw palmetto, as we said, has no contraindications, and will not interfere with sleeping pills, anxiety medications, or other drugs. It may even help them work. One of the reasons older men have problems sleeping at night is that their enlarged prostate wakes them up frequently to urinate. For them, one of the benefits of taking saw palmetto is that it reduces this frequency, which in itself may lead to better sleep and reduce the need for sleeping pills.

If the medication is prescribed, it is not a good idea to stop taking it without first checking with your doctor. Although medications are sometimes prescribed for more than one reason, sleeping pills are usually just for sleep, and if your sleeping does improve after taking saw palmetto, you might consider asking if you can reduce your medication. Doctors sometimes tell their patients that a pill is to help them sleep when it is really for something else and the doctor hopes it will also help sleep. For example, drugs that improve the function of your heart may also make it easier to sleep, so just be sure you know what you are taking, and why, before making any changes.

Taking Saw Palmetto without BPH

Research studies have not examined the question of whether saw palmetto is valuable as a preventive for prostate problems, but its action to reduce both DHT and estrogen hormone levels would seem to indicate its usefulness in prevention. And since you will not incur any risk by taking saw palmetto, it is probably a good idea to consider using it as preventive medicine. It doesn't cost very much, so that should not be an obstacle, and, again, there are no significant side effects.

The high numbers of men who end up with enlarged prostates argues in favor of doing everything possible to keep this from happening. This is especially true of men over age fifty, so starting to take saw palmetto in your forties is not unreasonable. As I said, I take small doses of saw palmetto regularly for prevention, and have done so for the past six years.

Proscar Risks Are Not Seen with Saw Palmetto

The drug finasteride (Proscar) has a history of possible problems for women who have any contact with its active ingredient, even if they are not taking the drug themselves. For example, a woman who gets pregnant while her partner is taking finasteride, or who comes into contact with the contents of the pills, may absorb enough of the drug herself to lead to birth defects in the urinary or genital organs of male fetuses. This may have given some people of childbearing age concern about this drug.

If a pregnant woman has contact with saw palmetto, however, there does not appear to be any risk to male offspring. Its beneficial effects on the hormones and enzymes do not seem to translate to side effects, even during pregnancy. There is no evidence of any side effects directly to the woman who contacts either finasteride or saw palmetto.

Saw Palmetto for Women

All the research I have seen on saw palmetto is for its value with prostate symptoms. However, there is also a history of its use in treating urinary tract disorders in both men and women. Saw palmetto has anti-inflammatory properties, which might help with painful urination and other symptoms of cystitis and urethritis (urinary tract infections). Since it is not an antibiotic, it would only help the symptoms, not eliminate a bacterial infection. (There are other herbs that might help with the infection: echinacea by enhancing immune function, or cranberry by preventing bacteria from attaching to the bladder lining.) For serious infections, of course, antibiotics may be necessary.

Saw palmetto may also help women with painful menstrual periods by relieving the spasms and cramps that often accompany their periods. Although these effects are not well documented, it could be that saw palmetto's beneficial effects on estrogen and testosterone hormones might contribute to these reported benefits.

CHAPTER 6

OTHER STEPS TO A HEALTHY PROSTATE

A s beneficial as it is, saw palmetto is only one of many dietary supplements that may help the prostate, and it is only part of a comprehensive program for prostate health. A complete program must also consider diet, lifestyle issues, and prevention of other prostate disorders besides benign enlargement, such as cancer.

Pygeum Africanum for Prostate

Pygeum africanum, an extract of an African tree bark, is another natural treatment for the prostate. It is a botanical supplement that helps relieve prostate symptoms and has research to prove it. In one study, although there were no changes in hormone levels in the blood of those who took pygeum, all of the evaluations showed improvement in the urinary symptoms and a reduction in the swelling of the prostate around the urethra. In another study done jointly in Austria, France, and Germany, the researchers found similar results, with highly significant improvement in BPH symptoms—the number of nighttime urinations, the residual urine volume, and the urine-flow rates all improved. And, as in the other studies, there were very few side effects, and these only minor.

In yet another study, with a placebo control, the researchers showed that, although many of the men improved with the placebo, there were significantly more that did well with the pygeum extract. The improvements were seen in the ease of starting urination, the frequency of nighttime urinations, and the sensation of incomplete emptying of the bladder.

Pygeum africanum
A botanical extract from an African tree bark that helps reduce the symptoms of BPH. It works well in combination with other herbs and nutrients.

Similar to other natural remedies for the prostate, all the pygeum studies indicate only a few minor side effects, although some experienced digestive upset. A comparison of saw palmetto and pygeum in one study showed that both were effective, but saw palmetto was somewhat better. The usual dose of Pygeum africanum is 25–50 mg of the standardized extract taken twice a day.

Combining Saw Palmetto and Pygeum

In the natural treatment of prostate enlargement, it is common to combine supplements that complement each other because, unlike many medications, nutrition and dietary supplements work well together and the results are even enhanced when taken in combination. Because nutrients work together in all cells, it is a good idea to combine different treatments unless there is a known negative interaction. There are no negative interactions when you take saw palmetto and pygeum together. Conversely, in most medical treatments, doctors and their patients are looking for some sort of magic bullet that will, all by itself, cure a problem with few, minor side effects. Unfortunately though, with most drugs, this is far from the typical result, and, unlike supplements, combining drugs can lead to serious adverse reactions.

Although there are only a few studies where

several natural treatments are combined, they have mostly shown that different supplements enhance the actions of the others. The health food stores have several combinations of herbs and nutrients that help the prostate, and if taken in combination, it may be possible that a lower dose of each of the combined supplements will help the prostate.

Other Herbs for the Prostate

At least one other herb has been helpful with prostate symptoms. Studies with extract of the stinging nettle plant (also called common nettle) have shown that it reduces prostate symptoms. Nettle may work by reducing the ability of DHT to bind to the sites where it is active, which results in less activity of this hormone, even though its amount remains unchanged.

In studies where it is combined with pygeum or saw palmetto, nettle extracts appear to enhance the action of each one. Although stinging nettles get their name from the stinging hairs on their stems and the leaves that cause a skin rash when you rub up against them, the extracts do not have any irritant effect. Nettle has been used as a food and a tea, and cooking eliminates its irritant properties. In fact, nettle extract has an anti-inflammatory effect, and among its other beneficial actions, it reduces allergy symptoms. The typical dose of nettle is 150–300 mg of standardized extract taken twice a day, but for allergies, a dose of 300 mg every three to four hours is sometimes recommended.

Other Natural Prostate Treatments

For many years, before saw palmetto or pygeum were commonly available as therapeutic supplements, nutritionally oriented doctors used other natural remedies for prostate enlargement with some success. One of the most widely used supplements for the prostate has historically been high doses of the trace mineral zinc. Zinc is important for many different body functions, such as antioxidant activity, immunity, the sense of taste and smell, wound healing, and managing the common cold. Some studies have shown that zinc lozenges can reduce the respiratory symptoms of a cold and cut short the duration of colds.

Zinc is particularly important for the normal functioning of the prostate. The prostate gland is very rich in zinc, with far more of it than any other organ in the body. It influences the hormones in the prostate, and, like saw palmetto, it can reduce the activity of the enzyme 5-alpha reductase, which promotes prostate enlargement. Small amounts of zinc are necessary for the activity of this enzyme, but higher levels appear to inhibit it.

It is also known that zinc levels are low in those who have either benign enlargement of the prostate or prostate cancer. In the past, physicians have recommended zinc in doses up to 150 mg per day for prostate enlargement. Recently, however, recommendations are to take 30–60 mg zinc *with* copper, to avoid an imbalance, as high doses of zinc can reduce the absorption of copper. Such high doses can also lower the good HDL cholesterol, which is not good. For this reason, I recommend the lower, but adequate, doses of zinc, along with the other effective treatments. In the context of a comprehensive program, this lower dose appears to be enough.

More Supplements for the Prostate

Numerous dietary supplements help the prostate, partly because they have either a direct effect on the prostate tissues, an indirect effect on hormone balance, or effects on other nutrients. For example, vitamin B_6, or pyridoxine, can help with the absorption of zinc, so the lower levels of zinc in the diet or in supplements may be more effective. Pyridoxine also helps to reduce the production of prolactin, a hormone produced in the pituitary gland, which stimulates milk production in lactating women. Prolactin also has an effect on the prostate because it promotes DHT production and, as a consequence, can stimulate the growth of prostate tissue. Reducing prolactin levels can help reduce the overgrowth of prostate tissue. Typical doses of pyridoxine are in the range of 50–200 mg per day. Very high doses, in excess of 500–2,000 mg, have been associated with peripheral neuropathy, a neurological disorder that includes loss of sensation, numbness, and tingling of the extremities, so it is wise to stay away from the highest doses.

Magnesium may be very important for symptoms of prostate enlargement, particularly the symptoms in the smooth muscles of the bladder, prostate tissue, and urethra. Magnesium helps to relax these involuntary muscles (those out of our conscious control). It is also important to take magnesium when you are taking extra vitamin B_6, because it helps to balance this nutrient. Typical doses of magnesium are from 300–1,000 mg daily. Magnesium aspartate, one of many forms found in any health food store, is one of the best-absorbed forms of this mineral. Magnesium is also very important for heart health and for the maintenance of normal blood pressure.

Similar to beta-carotene, lycopene is a red pigment in the carotenoid family of antioxidant nutrients that is found in pink grapefruit, tomatoes, and watermelon. High amounts of it in the diet or in supplements can protect the prostate from developing cancer, or can help in the treatment of prostate cancer if it does develop. Typical doses of a lycopene supplement range from 5–15 mg daily.

An herbal combination called PC-SPES has been shown to help reverse prostate cancer. It is a mixture that contains saw palmetto among a number of other less well-known herbs, and both research and my experience confirm that it is effective. Although it does have some side effects, such as breast enlargement and tenderness, it can clearly lower the PSA levels. When taking PC-SPES, I advise supervision by a nutritionally oriented practitioner. In 2001, some batches of PC-SPES were shown to contain hormones that were not on the label, and it has been removed from the market while further evaluations are done.

Amino Acids and Prostate Health

Amino acids are the building blocks of proteins. They get their name from a nitrogen-hydrogen combination called an amine, or amino group. There are eight essential amino acids, essential meaning the kind you must get in your diet because your body cannot manufacture them.

Generally, people get enough of the amino acids they need from the protein they eat. Most Americans, in fact, get too much protein, especially animal protein, so they have an abundance of amino acids. The amino acids from the diet go into manufacturing the different proteins of the body, or they are burned for energy, and any excess is converted to fat.

Some amino acids are also used for other purposes, such as providing the base molecule for the manufacture of hormones or nerve transmitters that carry the nerve signal from one nerve in a chain to the next one. Serotonin, for example, is a nerve transmitter derived from the amino acid tryptophan, and the hormone for the thyroid is derived from tyrosine, another amino acid.

Several reports suggest the value of certain amino acids in the treatment of prostate enlargement. The amino acids alanine, glutamic acid, and glycine were shown to reduce prostate symptoms in 70 to 90 percent (depending on which symptom was being evaluated) of the subjects in a study.

When amino acids are used for treatment, you cannot depend on getting them from food sources because other the amino acids present in protein drown out the therapeutic ones. To get the therapeutic levels, you need to take supplements. The recommended daily amounts vary from 50–200 mg for alanine, 200–1,000 mg for glutamic acid, and 200–400 mg for glycine.

Amino Acids
The building blocks of proteins. They get their name from a nitrogen-hydrogen combination called an amine, or amino group.

Fats and the Prostate

Depending on the kinds, and the balance in your diet and supplements, fats and oils can play a very important role in either maintaining prostate health or causing problems with the prostate. It is well known that too much fat or the wrong kind of fat in the diet is hazardous to your health in many ways. It is especially a problem when they are animal fats, or if the oils are hydrogenated (such as in margarine and shortening), or heavily processed (such as commercial vegetable oils).

Heating any oils during cooking increases the damage by oxidizing them and creating dangerous byproducts. Although polyunsaturated oils were heavily promoted for a time, they are exactly the ones that have the greatest likelihood of being oxidized by heat and light, and they increase the risk of cancer in many organs. When consuming any polyunsaturated oils, it is important to choose those that are minimally processed and not heated (look for labels that say cold-pressed). It is also important to take extra antioxidant nutrients, such as vitamins E and C, when you consume these oils.

Most people have too much fat in their diets, but not enough of the essential fatty acids (those that are required in the diet). Essential fatty acids influence hormone activity, immunity, inflammation, platelets, and smooth muscle action. In the right amounts, they are specifically valuable for prostate health. According to studies, men with BPH are deficient in essential fatty acids, and supplementing with them can help. I often recommend a combination of unrefined flaxseed oil for the omega-3 oils (one of the two essential fatty acids), and evening primrose oil or borage oil for gamma-linolenic acid (GLA), the source for the omega-6 oils (the other essential fatty acid).

Essential Fatty Acids
Beneficial dietary oils omega-3 and omega-6, called essential because they are required in the diet.

The dose of flaxseed oil is one to two tablespoons per day, and the dose of GLA is 240 mg (the equivalent of one borage oil capsule, or six evening primrose oil capsules). Certain fish, such as salmon and sardines, also contain an omega-3 oil called EPA. This oil is also available as a supplement in capsules or from cod liver oil. I recommend wild fish rather than farmed fish as much as possible, as the essential fatty acid composition is likely to be better. Alaskan salmon is always wild, as Alaska does not permit fish farming.

Dietary Habits and Prostate Health

As with almost every disease, lifestyle choices play

a role in the prevention and treatment of prostate disorders. This is especially true for preventing prostate cancer, but may also play an important role in prostate enlargement.

Try to choose a diet rich in vegetables, fresh fruits, whole grains, seeds, nuts, and beans. The more colorful the vegetable or fruit, the more likely it is to contain healthful nutrients. Eating meat has been shown to dramatically increase your risk of getting prostate cancer, and a vegetarian diet is healthier in many ways than one that includes meat. Also, avoid adding much oil of any kind to the diet. Although olive oil may not cause a problem, other oils and fats may be a serious risk, and it is no accident that, in places where the fat intake is low, there is also a low incidence of prostate cancer. (Black Africans who are native have a low incidence of prostate cancer and a low-fat diet, while African-Americans have a high incidence of prostate cancer and a high fat intake.) The foods I have recommended here provide a diet that is high in fiber, low in fat, and rich in phytonutrients and flavonoids, all of which are protective.

Read ingredient labels carefully and avoid foods that contain added sugar and artificial or synthetic additives, such as colors, flavorings, preservatives, and sweeteners. These do nothing to enhance health, and are usually present only in heavily processed foods that you don't need in your diet anyway.

Avoid caffeine and alcohol as much as possible. Caffeine has been associated with fibrocystic breast disease, and since the breast contains glandular and fibrous tissue like the prostate, it is possible that caffeine may also cause problems for the prostate. It is also a diuretic, and increases the frequency of urination, which is already a problem for men with BPH. Alcohol affects the hormones that play a role in prostate enlargement, and it is best to keep alcohol intake low. Liver damage from excess alcohol consumption leads to increases in estrogen levels, because the liver is the organ that breaks down these hormones, and if it is damaged, it cannot do its job properly.

Specific Foods to Prevent Prostate Cancer

Several specific foods are even more beneficial than the general guidelines above. Include some soybean products in your diet, such as soymilk or tofu. Natural hormonelike isoflavone substances in soy (called phytoestrogens) help to prevent cancer of the prostate and many other organs. If you think you don't like tofu, you may be surprised to learn that it is commonly used in fried rice dishes in Chinese restaurants where it is disguised by the other ingredients. Most people find they do like it if it is prepared correctly. Other forms of soy products are tempeh, a fermented soybean cake common in Indonesia, and soy protein powders that can be added to fruit smoothies, other blender drinks, or even vegetable stews. However, avoid the highly processed soy-derived products such as texturized vegetable protein (TVP) and the many imitation foods made from it, including some vegetable broths and imitation chicken and meat.

Whole grains have also been shown to decrease cancer risks. In population studies, those who have the highest intake of whole grains have a lower incidence of cancer for almost every cancer studied, including prostate. This means it is important to include whole grains in the diet, such as barley, brown rice, corn, millet, oatmeal, rye, whole wheat, and several others. On the other hand, refined grains, such as white flour products, are associated with increasing risks of disease, including cancer and heart disease, so it is best to avoid them altogether.

Nutrients That Help the Prostate

As previously mentioned, lycopene is in the carotene family of vitamins (beta-carotene is the best-known carotenoid, being the orange color found in carrots, but there are many other nutritious carotenoids). Lycopene is found in pink grapefruit, tomatoes, and watermelon, and it is also available as a supplement. Research shows that tomatoes can reduce the risk of prostate cancer, probably because of the lycopene they contain. We know that men whose diets are high in lycopene have a lower chance of getting prostate cancer than men with lower levels of lycopene intake. Any tomato product is beneficial, from fresh tomatoes, to tomato sauce, to tomato juice, with the highest amounts of lycopene found in tomatoes that have been concentrated by cooking. You can also take 5–15 mg lycopene supplements to make sure you get enough.

Garlic contains a number of substances that are protective. Whether taken as a food or a supplement, it is associated with a lower chance of getting prostate cancer. Garlic is widely available in a deodorized supplement for those who don't like garlic, or don't wish to smell of it every day. (I personally like it a lot, I eat it often, and it is a common ingredient in many of the ethnic foods I enjoy.) Supplements of deodorized garlic contain about 500 mg of concentrated extract. You might take two to four of these a day if you are not eating garlic regularly.

Selenium is a trace mineral that protects

against many cancers. It works with vitamins C and E as a free-radical scavenger. Selenium is low in the diets of most people, mainly because of selenium-depleted soil, but it is readily available as an inexpensive supplement. Typical supplemental doses range from 100-400 mcg (micrograms) a day (a microgram is one thousandth of a milligram).

Lifestyle Habits and Prostate Health

As with almost any health issue, it is important to get regular exercise, such as bicycling, jogging, skating, skiing, walking, or using exercising machines—ski machines, stair machines, and treadmills are examples. Exercise stimulates our immunity and eliminates toxins. There are specific exercises that help urinary control. Known as Kegel exercises, they consist of contracting the muscles around the rectal area as though you are trying to stop urination or a bowel movement, and doing them many times a day may help in bladder control.

Regular exercise reduces prostate symptoms. Try to do at least thirty minutes of exercise most days. When people ask me if they have to exercise every day, I ask them, "How often does a gorilla exercise?" The answer, of course, is every time they want to eat or play, which is more than once a day. This may be too much to fit into your schedule (gorillas don't have to sit at a desk and work), but there is consensus that exercising at least four to six times a week is beneficial. It has even been associated with a decreased risk of cancer and heart disease. (And, as another peripheral benefit, recent findings suggest that exercise contributes to weight loss more than any diet.)

If you have not been doing exercise regularly,

start with just ten or fifteen minutes of walking and increase your time by a few minutes a week. It is easy to determine how fast to go, because you should not get out of breath during the exercise, but you should work up a sweat by the time you get to thirty minutes. You don't need a formal exercise program if you keep very active by gardening, mowing the lawn, walking or bicycling on your errands, and taking stairs instead of elevators when possible. However, most people tend to miss out on exercise unless they make specific exercise a part of their routines.

Other Lifestyle Habits in Prostate Health

The placebo effect demonstrates that our emotional state, thought processes, and expectations are components of most illnesses. They lead to both the feeling of improvement and an actual measurable improvement, but if they can influence illness for the better, they can also be involved in causing, or worsening, symptoms. Stress is particularly damaging. It increases general health risks in many ways, including its role in increasing the output of the adrenal hormones, the metabolism, and the damaging oxidation by - products. Practicing a stress-reduction technique can be very helpful in reducing cancer risks, and with health in general.

Five or six times a day, you should try to do some breathing exercises, stretching, or yoga, or simply close your eyes and imagine your favorite place for about three or four minutes. You might consider reading about meditation, or getting some help learning how to do it. Whatever relaxation method works for you is fine.

Finally, I can't say enough about the dangers of tobacco smoke, even the second-hand smoke that most of us find hard to avoid. It is probably one of the most dangerous substances we humans expose ourselves to voluntarily. It leads to many cancers, and puts an enormous burden on our normal protective mechanisms. Smoking also appears to increase the risk of developing BPH. Avoid it!

CHAPTER 7

SEXUAL FUNCTION AND MEN'S HEALTH

Healthy sexual functioning is a pleasure that can be enjoyed until very late in life. However, many unhealthy habits and practices can adversely influence the ability to maintain this function. Although many men equate the prostate with their sexual functioning, an enlarged prostate (BPH) doesn't need to affect your sexual function at all. Sexual dysfunction, or erectile dysfunction (a better term than impotence), is a significant issue for men as they age, but it is not necessarily related to problems with the prostate. Good nutrition, hormonal balance, physical fitness, and stress can all contribute to your normal sexual functioning, and they are all in your control.

BPH and Sex Drive

Benign prostatic hyperplasia does not affect your libido (sex drive), your ability to have an erection, or your ability to have normal orgasms and ejaculations. If you are taking saw palmetto for your enlarged prostate symptoms, it not only has no harmful side effects in relation to sexual functioning, it has even been used to enhance libido and potency.

If you have an infection or an inflammation of the prostate (prostatitis) that leads to painful or uncomfortable urination, it may temporarily decrease your desire or sexual function. This should clear up after proper treatment of the infection. While being treated, it is a good idea to take dietary supplements that may help reduce the inflammation and speed your recovery from the infection.

Early prostate cancer is also not a problem, but in the later stages, or after treatment with surgery, radiation, or drugs, there can sometimes be interference with sexual functioning. Depending on the treatment, however, this is often not a permanent problem. Even if you have surgery to remove your prostate, it is still possible to have an active sex life. Although this is not always the case, you should be aware that the prostate is not essential to the desire or the ability to have sex.

Remember that prostate enlargement is extremely widespread, and it should not interfere with your sexual pleasure. There are many natural treatments available to help you avoid the side effects of drugs and surgery, and they all can help you feel good about yourself, in spite of having an enlarged prostate, or even prostate cancer. Sexual activity, in fact, is probably helpful in maintaining the health of the prostate.

Lifestyle and Sexual Functioning

A number of lifestyle choices play a role in healthy sexuality. Alcohol consumption, lack of exercise, obesity, and poor nutrition in general can decrease both your libido and your sexual functioning. The diet I recommended earlier for the healthy prostate is the same diet I recommend here for optimum sexual functioning: one that is high in vegetables, fruits, whole grains, beans, seeds, nuts, fish, and organic eggs. Losing weight (and 75 percent of Americans are overweight) requires you to avoid fatty or fried foods, hydrogenated oils, processed foods containing artificial ingredients, sugar, and white flour, as well as overeating any foods. These choices are also good for your overall health.

Regular consumption of alcohol, beyond a small amount, can lead to a deterioration in your sexual function, probably due in part to its effects on your hormones and your liver. Too much alcohol at any one time can have an immediate negative effect on the ability to achieve and maintain an erection. The evidence that red wine may be good for your heart is still controversial (heart disease is still the leading cause of death in France), and, so far, there is no reliable evidence that a healthy non-drinker in middle age should take up drinking to improve health.

Many studies have shown that exercise helps your health. You don't have to be a competitive athlete to benefit, and you don't have to exhaust yourself to be healthy. A simple plan of regular, repetitive motion, such as bicycling, jogging, rollerblading, skiing, swimming, using exercise machines, or just plain walking, is beneficial. If you do twenty to forty minutes of repetitive-motion exercise four to five times a week, you will be in shape in no time. You can exercise without getting out of breath, but do try to work up a sweat. This simple guideline should keep you at aerobic levels of exercise. If there is no exercise you love, get an exercise machine and work out while watching the news or reading a magazine.

Exercise will give you more energy, improve your digestion and elimination, your psychological well-being, and your sleep. If you can add some muscle-building exercise, such as elastic resistance bands or light weights, it would further improve your health. Increasing your muscle mass improves your insulin regulation and your sugar metabolism and, by burning calories, your ability to control your weight. Doing this for fifteen to twenty minutes three times a week would be a good start.

Health Conditions and Sexuality

If you have hardening of the arteries (atherosclerosis), and you have problems with erectile dysfunction, this could be due to poor circulation through the arteries to the penis. With the standard American diet (SAD), plaque in the arteries starts in the teen years, and without changing your diet, this will build up over the years, leading to a closure of your arteries, and contributing to the problem. It also leads to heart disease, another contributor to sexual dysfunction.

Diabetes, increasingly prevalent now, leads to two problems that play a role in sexual functioning: it increases hardening of the arteries, and it causes diabetic peripheral neuropathy, which is a decreased ability of the long nerves to carry impulses. This problem leads to numbness and tingling, and a loss of sensitivity in the nerves that is essential to normal erections.

Other health conditions, such as chronic back pain, a low thyroid, neurological diseases, or psychiatric disorders, can also lead to sexual dysfunction. It is essential that you get a complete medical evaluation is to find out whether atherosclerosis, diabetes, or any of these conditions are part of the problem.

Supplements Help Sexual Function

While many supplements can contribute to general health, and the management of back pain, diabetes, heart disease, neuropathy, and psychiatric disorders, some specific supplements may be helpful with erectile dysfunction.

Normal erections require the presence of nitric

oxide, a substance made by the cells lining the arteries that is essential for the muscles of the blood vessels to relax and open up the blood flow. In fact, nitric oxide was called the endothelial-derived relaxing factor before it was chemically identified. This blood flow is necessary for engorgement of the penile erectile tissue. The cells make nitric oxide from the amino acid L-arginine, and taking supplements of L-arginine has been helpful with erectile dysfunction. The typical dose of L-arginine is 2,000–8,000 mg at one time, shortly before sexual activity. It may also help to take it regularly, in a dose of 1,000–2,000 mg daily. L-arginine should be balanced with some extra L-lysine, as some experts believe that an excess of arginine makes a person more prone to the development of herpes viruses.

Another supplement that helps with blood flow through the small blood vessels is ginkgo biloba. Ginkgo extract contains protective antioxidant flavonoids that also help circulation by inhibiting the platelet activity that can slow circulation. It also contains substances called terpenes that increase circulation and protect the nervous system. These benefits of ginkgo for the nervous tissue and circulation may make it beneficial for erectile dysfunction. The usual dose is 120–240 mg per day of the standardized extract containing 24 percent flavones and 6 percent terpene compounds.

The herb yohimbe has been successfully used in the treatment of erectile dysfunction. Its active component is yohimbine, an indole alkaloid that dilates blood vessels. Since yohimbe does have potential side effects, such as anxiety, increased blood pressure, and a rapid heart rate, it is a good idea to consult with a nutritionally oriented practitioner before taking this herb. And, if you have kidney or liver disease, you should avoid taking yohimbe. The typical dose is 15–30 mg of the standardized extract.

Taking chromium supplements in relatively high doses enhances the action of insulin, and can help with sugar control in diabetes. Research shows that those with type II diabetes who take 1,000 mcg of chromium per day can reduce their blood sugars to normal 50 percent of the time, and in 90 percent of the cases, they can help people come off their medications. Chromium also helps control lipids in the blood.

Another supplement that helps people with diabetes is alpha-lipoic acid. This is an antioxidant that works in both the water- and lipid-based tissues, and it is particularly good for the nerves and the brain. Doses from 100–300 mg daily can help control blood sugars and 1,000 mg daily is helpful for peripheral neuropathy.

CHAPTER 8

HEART DISEASE AND MEN'S HEALTH

Although heart disease due to atherosclerosis (hardening of the arteries) is the leading cause of death for both men and women, it is often thought of as a men's disease. Perhaps this is because, prior to menopause, it is much less common in women. (When all age groups are tested, heart disease is the leading killer of women.) In developed countries, heart disease starts in youth, largely because of diet, and later, because of the diet combined with the sedentary lifestyle that most people lead. Heart disease is almost always the result of lifestyle choices that can be changed with a little education, effort, and motivation.

Atherosclerotic Heart Disease and Lifestyle

Atherosclerotic (also called arteriosclerotic) diseases result from a buildup of plaque (fatty, fibrous, calcified deposits) in the arterial wall, which reduces and eventually blocks the blood flow to the vital organs. The damage to the arteries results from free-radical injury and inflammation, both of which can be related to lifestyle choices. Common symptoms of heart disease include chest tightness or pain, which may be felt in the left arm, the back, or the jaw, shortness of breath, and fatigue. The chest symptoms may also be perceived as a sensation of pressure, like an elephant sitting on your chest, as heartburn, or simply as indigestion. Some of the recent tests to predict the risks of heart disease are related to inflammation.

The lifestyle modifications that are the most important for helping to prevent and treat heart disease are dietary changes and exercise, with stress management and dietary supplements also playing vital roles in reducing the problem. Heart disease is not simply genetic. When we see that American teenagers between the ages of fifteen and nineteen already have plaque in their arteries, we cannot blame it on genetics. It is almost certainly related to their diets and their lack of exercise. In the Korean War, doctors examined young American soldiers who died of trauma, and they already had plaque in their arteries, while the young Koreans did not. But when Koreans move to the United States and eat the Western diet, they too develop the same arterial diseases. As fast foods and heavily processed fatty and sugary foods spread around the world, we see in their wake preventable increases in diabetes, heart disease, hypertension, obesity, and other degenerative diseases.

Atherosclerosis
The gradual buildup of plaque in the arterial wall, which reduces, and eventually blocks, the flow of blood to the vital organs.

Diet Changes for Better Health

This diet is the same one I recommended above for the prostate and for sexual function. Cut down on artificial flavors, colors, preservatives, and sweeteners, processed foods, white flour, and sugar, all of which are junk, not food. Reduce animal products in the diet, except for fish, which is beneficial because of the essential fatty acids they contain. Meat, chicken, and dairy products, especially fatty ones, contribute to increased mortality from heart disease and cancer. In fact, mortality from all diseases is lower in vegetarians than non-vegetarians. Eat more fresh vegetables, fruits, whole grains, beans, seeds, and nuts. Numerous scientific studies come to this same conclusion, and they come from the evaluation of many different populations all over the world.

There are any number of fad diets that claim to be helpful in losing weight. They may lead to weight loss because they reduce caloric intake, but they are not healthful diets. The so-called value of the high-protein and high-fat diets is not supported by the medical literature. Just the opposite, in fact, because they are associated with more arthritis, cancer, diabetes, gallstones, gout, heart disease, and osteoporosis. These diets have little fiber, an important dietary component, and they are low in protective phytochemicals and bioflavonoids (healthful plant pigments).

If you eat dairy products, choose low fat, organic sources, and try to eat only organic eggs, preferably those from chickens fed omega-3 oils, if these are available. Although I used to recommend mainly salmon, the farming of fish is now widespread, and not many fish farms use natural methods. As a result, the good essential fatty acid composition of the fish is altered. The growth hormone that is used to double the growth rate of the fish is untested for its health effects, and both infections and the use of antibiotics in fish farming are increasing. In order to avoid these problems, I now suggest sardines (water packed) as the preferred source, or Alaskan salmon (Alaska does not permit fish farming). You don't need much animal product in the diet, but I believe it is beneficial to have some, and small amounts of fish, low-fat organic yogurt, or organic eggs are the best sources.

Exercise for the Heart

Please review the exercise program described above. It is critically important for both prevention and treatment of heart disease. Of course, if you already have heart disease, you must pay attention to the intensity of your exercise, so you don't develop symptoms, such as chest pain or tightness, lightheadedness, palpitations, or shortness of breath.

Supplements for Preventing Heart Disease

I always recommend starting with a high-potency, multivitamin-mineral combination. This should give you the B-complex (50–100 mg), some vitamins C and E, calcium and magnesium (500 mg each), and trace minerals. However, no multivitamin preparation has everything you need in adequate doses, so you do need to take some extra supplements for greater protection.

For example, take extra vitamins C and E. They act as potent antioxidants, protecting the blood vessels from free-radical damage. These vitamins also help to lower cholesterol while raising the good HDL cholesterol. I usually recommend about 4,000 mg of vitamin C and 400 IU of vitamin E. If your multiple has this amount of E, then it may be enough until you are over age forty, when you might want to take an extra 400–800 IU. I advise using only the natural d-alpha tocopherol (as opposed to dl-alpha), plus the mixed tocopherols (beta, gamma, and delta, and especially the gamma, which is being increasingly studied for its benefits).

Selenium is a trace mineral that is associated

with less heart disease (and less cancer). Along with other antioxidants, it works as a component of the enzyme glutathione peroxidase, which boosts the activity of vitamin E. Usually 200–400 mcg per day is a good dose. The same daily 200–400 mcg dose of chromium contributes to preventing heart disease because chromium helps control blood sugar (diabetes is a risk factor for heart disease), and it promotes normal blood fat and cholesterol. Folic acid and vitamin B_{12} help to lower homocysteine levels, and homocysteine, an amino acid in the blood, has been found to damage arteries and lead to increased atherosclerosis. While many supplements are useful in preventing heart disease, some of them are particularly important for treatment if you already have heart disease.

Coenzyme Q_{10} and Heart Disease

Coenzyme Q_{10} (CoQ_{10}) is essential for the production of energy in the membranes of the tiny mitochondria engines in every cell. It is needed for the conversion of fatty acids to the energy molecule called ATP. CoQ_{10} is especially abundant in heart muscle, and it is an excellent antioxidant. Some studies have found it to be about four times more potent than vitamin E. CoQ_{10} supplements can help alleviate angina, arrhythmias, congestive heart failure, high blood pressure, and shortness of breath. CoQ_{10} also increases exercise tolerance. Side benefits of taking CoQ_{10} are antioxidant protection from the free-radical damage associated with aging, improved immunity, and increased energy levels in general.

Antioxidants
Protective substances that prevent damage to cells, membranes, molecules, and tissues from excessive exposure to hazardous molecules called free radicals.

Although CoQ_{10} is not really a vitamin because your body makes it, the amount your body makes declines with age and illness. The typical dose for treatment of heart disease is 100–400 mg daily, depending on the severity of the problem. For prevention, I think it is a good idea to take 50–100 mg a day, especially if you are over age forty, if you have any other illness, or if you have a family history of heart disease.

L-Carnitine and Heart Disease

Another supplement that helps the heart is L-carnitine. This derivative of amino acids is essential for transporting fatty acids across the membranes of the mitochondria where they are used for energy production (because of this, it works well with CoQ_{10}, and they are commonly taken together). When there is pain due to a lack of oxygen in the heart muscle (angina), the level of L-carnitine drops dramatically, and the heart muscle switches to glucose metabolism instead of fat. As a result, more lactic acid is produced, and this makes the pain worse. If there is enough L-carnitine available in advance, the pain is lessened, and the like - lihood of damage to the heart is reduced. Although you normally produce L-carnitine, as with some other essential substances, the production declines with age. Supplements of L-carnitine are typically in the range of 500–1,000 mg twice a day. Some athletes take even more to enhance their stamina.

Botanical Supplements for the Heart

Garlic has been used for millennia, not only as a culinary delight, but also as a therapeutic dietary supplement. It helps the heart in many ways. It reduces your blood pressure, which is a risk factor for the development of heart disease. Garlic supplements also reduce the adhesiveness (stickiness) of platelets, reducing the possibility of excessive clotting inside the blood vessels.

Garlic reduces total cholesterol levels while increasing the good HDL cholesterol, so it helps in both prevention and treatment. As a free-radical scavenger, garlic helps prevent the oxidative reactions that promote atherosclerosis. It appears to protect the enzymes in the cells lining the arteries. These are the cells that produce nitric oxide, the molecule essential for relaxation of the blood vessels, and garlic appears to promote the production of this vital substance. Additionally, garlic acts as an antibiotic and antiviral substance, it can enhance immunity, and it can reduce the incidence of some cancers, all without side effects.

I recommend eating garlic as part of the diet, and supplementing for treatment. The usual dose of garlic is 500–1,500 mg twice a day. If you use deodorized garlic, you can take your garlic every day without fear of being ostracized socially.

Hawthorn berry is a valuable herb that has been used for centuries for the heart. Its active components include several flavonoid pigments, and it improves the strength of the heart muscle, and relaxes the blood vessels, allowing for improved blood flow. Hawthorn berry supplements can improve exercise capacity, and can mildly reduce elevated blood pressure in people with congestive heart failure. The usual dose of standardized hawthorn extract is 250–500 mg twice a day.

I mentioned ginkgo biloba earlier for the circulation benefits it provides. Those same effects make it useful in heart disease, and it is commonly taken in the same doses, 60–120 mg of standardized extract, twice a day.

Amino Acids for Heart Disease

L-taurine, an amino acid, helps to increase the strength of the heart muscle and reduces the overactivity of the fibers that conduct the impulse for the heartbeat. For people with congestive heart failure, L-taurine supplements are safe and effective additions to their treatment, and they may also reduce arrhythmias. In animal studies, taurine has been shown to be helpful in controlling blood pressure. The typical dose is 500–1,000 mg twice a day.

Earlier I mentioned L-arginine as a precursor to nitric oxide, the blood-vessel relaxant. For this same reason, it is helpful in heart disease. In doses of 1,000–6,000 mg daily, it improves angina, heart failure, hypertension, and immune function, as well as sexual function.

L-Lysine reduces the tendency of blood-lipid components to stick to artery walls and release deposits of damaging lipoprotein(a). The usual dose is about 1,500 mg daily for treatment.

Relaxation and the Heart

Putting together a complete program for prevention or treatment must include more than diet, exercise, and supplements. Stress management is also an important therapy for almost any health condition, including cancer, heart disease, and sexual functioning. I always recommend some form of relaxation for all my heart patients, and there are many that work well. I would also recommend that you practice breathing exercises, laughter, various forms of meditation, and visualization to reduce your stress responses. Norman Cousins, the author of *Anatomy of an Illness*, also wrote *The Healing Heart* about his recovery from a serious heart attack, using laughter and other healthful practices, and emphasizing the power-ful role that our minds play in healing.

I also recommend that you look into chelation therapy for heart disease. This is a very safe intra-venous treatment with a synthetic amino acid that binds with calcium and heavy metals, such as lead, and removes them from the body. Chelation therapy has been done since the 1950s, but it re-mains controversial. In spite of this, the number of doctors who are doing chelation is increasing. Doctors in the American College for Advance-ment in Medicine usually administer this therapy, and you can find a doctor in your area by looking at their website (see page 78).

CONCLUSION

Prostate health is only one of the issues that men face as they age, and most of them can be influenced by diet and lifestyle. Saw palmetto is a part of a comprehensive program to take care of your prostate. Similar health programs can prevent and treat sexual dysfunction and heart disease, the leading cause of death in the United States and other Western countries, and they not only help with the prostate, sexual functioning, and heart disease, but also with almost any health problem, in the process giving you some measure of control over your own care.

Your own practitioner may be very willing to participate with you in this kind of care, because many of them are becoming aware of their patients' interest in more natural remedies, and increasing numbers of them are beginning to get trained in complementary and alternative medicine. If your doctor is unwilling to consider using saw palmetto or other dietary supplements, perhaps you should give him or her a copy of this book, or go to another practitioner who is more versed in alternative/complementary methods.

No matter what your health problems, consider all the options and make informed decisions about the kind of care that you want. If you can't find a doctor who will work with you in this form of treatment, you can call the American College for

Advancement in Medicine (ACAM) at 1-800-532-3688 to locate a doctor in your area who is open to innovative treatments. You can also look them up online at www.acam.org.

Using natural remedies as part of your comprehensive healthcare program for both treatment and prevention is a positive step in the changing healthcare picture. As more conventional doctors become aware of these treatments and add them to their medical skills, you will find it easier to get the medical help you want. Today, the American population is doing this more than ever before, and you would do well to join them. It will help you, your family, and anyone who learns from your example.

SELECTED
REFERENCES

Adriazola Semino, M, Lozano Ortega, JL, Garcia Cobo, E, et al. Symptomatic treatment of benign hypertrophy of the prostate. Comparative study of prazosin and serenoa repens. *Archivas Espanol Urologia*, 1992; 45(3):211–3.

Barlet, A, Albrecht, J, Aubert, A, et al. Efficacy of Pygeum africanum extract in the medical therapy of urination disorders due to benign prostatic hyperplasia: evaluation of objective and subjective parameters. A placebo-controlled double-blind multicenter study. *Wien Klinische Wochenschrift*, 1990; 102(22):667–73.

Bogden, JD, Oleske, JM, Lavenhar, MA, et al. Effects of one year of supplementation with zinc and other micronutrients on cellular immunity in the elderly. *Journal of the American College of Nutrition*, 1990; 9(3):214–25.

Braeckman, J. The extract of Serenoa repens in the treatment of benign prostatic hyperplasia: a multicenter open study. *Current Therapy Research*, 1994; 55:776–85.

Carani, C, Salvioli, V, Scuteri, A, et al. Urological and sexual evaluation of treatment of benign prostatic disease using Pygeum africanum at high doses. *Archivas Italiano Urologia Nefrologia e Andrologia*, 1991; 63(3):341–5.

Champault, G, Bonnard, AM, Cauquil, J, Patel, JC. Actualite Therapeutique: The medical treatment of prostatic adenoma. *Annals of Urology* (Paris), 1984; 18(6):407-10.

Champault, G, Patel, JC, Bonnard, AM. A double-blind trial of an extract of the plant Serenoa repens in benign prostatic hyperplasia. *British Journal of Clinical Pharmacology*, 1984; 18(3): 461–2.

Chatenoud, L, Tavani, A, La Vecchia, C, et al. Whole grain food intake and cancer risk. *International Journal of Cancer*, 1998; 77(1):24–8.

Dufour, B, Choquenet, C, Revol, M, Faure, G, Jorest, R. Controlled study of the effects of Pygeum africanum extract on the functional symptoms of prostatic adenoma. *Annals of Urology* (Paris), 1984; 18(3):193–5.

Flamm, J, Kiesswetter, H. A urodynamic study of patients with benign prostatic hypertrophy treated conservatively with phytotherapy or testosterone. *Wien Klinische Wochenschrift*, 1979; 91 (18):622–7.

Food Drug Cosmetic Law Reports, New Developments, 1990; 1427:42,434–41.

Gerber, GS, Zagaja, GP, Bales, GT, Chodak, GW, Contreras, BA. Saw palmetto (Serenoa repens) in men with lower urinary tract symptoms: effects on urodynamic parameters and voiding symptoms. *Urology*, 1998; 51(6):1003–7.

Grasso, M, Montesano, A, Buonaguidi, A, et al. Comparative effects of alfuzosin versus Serenoa repens in the treatment of symptomatic benign prostatic hyperplasia. *Archivas Espanol Urologia*, 1995; 48(1):97–103.

Habib, FK, Hammond, GL, Lee, IR, et al. Metal-androgen interrelationships in carcinoma and hyperplasia of the human prostate. *Journal of Endocrinology,* 1976; 71(1):133–41.

Hayes RB, Ziegler RG, Gridley G, et al. Dietary factors and risks for prostate cancer among blacks and whites in the United States. *Cancer Epidemiology Biomarkers and Prevention,* 1999; 8(1): 25–34.

Keen, CL, Gershwin, ME. Zinc deficiency and immune function. *Annual Review of Nutrition,* 1990; 10:415–31.

Kortt, MA, Bootman, JL. The economics of benign prostatic hyperplasia treatment: a literature review. *Clinical Therapeutics,* 1996; 18(6):1227–41.

Krzeski, T, Kazon, M, Borkowski, A, Witeska, A, Kuczera, J. Combined extracts of Urtica dioica and Pygeum africanum in the treatment of benign prostatic hyperplasia: double-blind comparison of two doses. *Clinical Therapeutics,* 1993; 15(6): 1011–20.

Mossad, SB, Macknin, ML, Medendorp, SV, Mason, P. Zinc gluconate lozenges for treating the common cold. A randomized, double-blind, placebo-controlled study. *Annals of Internal Medicine,* 1996; 125(2):81–8.

Pfeifer, BL, Pirani, JF, Hamann, SR, Klippel, KF. PC-SPES, a dietary supplement for the treatment of hormone-refractory prostate cancer. *British Journal of Urology International,* 2000; 85(4):481–5.

Platz, EA, Kawachi, I, Rimm, EB, et al. Physical activity and benign prostatic hyperplasia. *Archives of Internal Medicine,* 1998; 158(21):2349–56.

Platz, EA, Rimm, EB, Kawachi, I, et al. Alcohol consumption, cigarette smoking, and risk of benign prostatic hyperplasia. *American Journal of Epidemiology,* 1999; 149(2):106–15.

Plosker, GL, Brogden, RN. Serenoa repens (Permixon). A review of its pharmacology and therapeutic efficacy in benign prostatic hyperplasia. *Drugs & Aging,* 1996; (5):379–95.

Schneider, HJ, Honold, E, Masuhr, T. Treatment of benign prostatic hyperplasia. Results of a treatment study with the phytogenic combination of Sabal extract WS 1473 and Urtica extract WS 1031 in urologic specialty practices. *Fortschrift Medizinische,* 1995; 113(3):37–40.

Wynder, EL, Rose, DP, Cohen, LA. Nutrition and prostate cancer: a proposal

for dietary intervention, *Nutrition and Cancer,* 1994; 22(1): 1–9.

OTHER BOOKS
AND RESOURCES

Janson, Michael. *Dr. Janson's New Vitamin Revolution*. New York, NY: Penguin-Putnam-Avery, 2000.

Murray, Michael, Pizzorno, Joseph. *Encyclopedia of Natural Medicine*. Rocklin, CA: Prima Publishing, 1991.

Schachter, Michael. *The Natural Way to a Healthy Prostate*. New Canaan, CT: Keats Publishing, 1995.

Werbach, Melvin, Murray, Michael. *Botanical Influences on Illness*. Tarzana, CA: Third Line Press, 1994.

GreatLife Magazine
Consumer magazine with articles on vitamins, minerals, herbs, and foods.
Available for free at many health and natural food stores.

Physical Magazine
Magazine oriented to body builders and other serious athletes.

Customer service:
1-800-676-4333
P.O. Box 74908
Los Angeles, CA 90004
Subscriptions: 12 issues per year, $19.95 in the U.S.; $31.95 outside the U.S.

The Nutrition Reporter™ newsletter

Monthly newsletter that summarizes recent medical research on vitamins, minerals, and herbs.

Customer service:

P.O. Box 30246

Tucson, AZ 85751-0246

e-mail: jack@thenutritionreporter.com

www.nutritionreporter.com

Subscriptions: $26 per year (12 issues) in the U.S.; $32 U.S. or $48 CNC for Canada; $38 for other countries

Dr. Michael Janson's Website:
www.drjanson.com

Updates of the medical literature; editorials; answers to commonly asked questions, or individual questions of general interest; free monthly newsletter available by e-mail.

American College for Advancement in Medicine
www.acam.org

Information about conferences in complementary and alternative medicine and a referral source if you are looking for doctors who practice this medicine.

INDEX

ACAM. *See* American College for Advancement in Medicine.

Aging, 6, 18, 26

Alanine, 53

Alaskan salmon, 54, 69

Alcohol, 55–56, 63

Alpha-lipoic acid, 66

American College for Advancement in Medicine, 75, 77–78

American Urological Association Symptom Index, 10

Amino acids, 24, 52–53

Angina, 72

Antioxidants, 66, 70, 71

Atherosclerosis, 64, 67–68

Benign prostatic hyperplasia, 6–12, 18, 22–26, 47–56, 62
  causes of, 18
  diagnostic tests for, 10–12
  evaluation of, 9–10
  sex drive and, 62–63
  symptoms, 7–10, 24–25, 26
  treatment, 13–16, 22, 23–26, 47–56

Benign prostatic hypertrophy. *See* Benign prostatic hyperplasia.

Bladder, emptying of, 8, 32

Blood pressure, 72

Borage oil, 54

Botanical medicine, 23, 34–35, 47–54, 77–78

Boyarsky Index, 9–10

BPH. *See* Benign prostatic hyperplasia.

British Journal of Urology, 15

Caffeine, 55

Chelation therapy, 75

Cholesterol, 70, 73

Chromium, 66, 71

Coenzyme Q_{10}, 71–72

Colds, 50

Common nettle. *See* Stinging nettle.

Control groups, 28

Printed in the USA
CPSIA information can be obtained
at www.ICGtesting.com
JSHW012009140824
68134JS00004B/88